# Inside Her (Mind): Secrets of the Female Psyche to Attract Women, Keep Them Seduced, and Bulletproof Your Relationship

## By Patrick King

### Dating and Image Coach at
www.PatrickKingConsulting.com

# Inside Her (Mind): Secrets of the Female Psyche to Attract Women, Keep Them Seduced, and Bulletproof Your Relationship

## Introduction

1. Being assertive isn't being an asshole.

2. Tarzan usually leads.

3. No time machines allowed during arguments.

4. Men can be "crazy" too.

5. Make it safe for her to be vulnerable.

6. Match up your styles of affection.

7. Compromise, don't sacrifice.

8. ~~Why can't you be more like Alison?~~

9. Really, her favorite bands are a dealbreaker?

10. Rationalization is usually a cover.

11. Who loves you the most? You!

12. Inspire her, motivate her.

13. The only "The One" questions you'll need.

14. Day to day chemistry beats the rich yoga instructor.

15. "Maybe" is usually "I'm scared to actually say no."

16. Relationship pants are meant for two.

17. Let her feminine qualities shine.

# Introduction

A relationship exists in many phases, and it's not always clear which one we're in. After all, it's not like we get a badge every time we advance to the next stage like we're Boy Scouts.

We start out with the mystery, allure, and chase of a new partner. This is exciting, thrilling, and it's the stuff that movies are made about. Palms sweating, butterflies in the stomach... yup, that's the good stuff. Every text from them is a moment of triumph, and your mind is a hamster on his wheel every night that you don't see them.

Let's call this the Chase phase.

Next, after you discover that your affections are returned and that there's the potential for something real between you and the other person, you quickly dip into the "I can't get enough of you" mindset. You fight the urge to spend every waking second together, and start showing up to events and activities together enough so that people always ask where your partner is when you're alone.

You'll go out of your way to pick up that muffin that your partner really loves, and celebrate any milestone possible. Friends, activities, and hobbies fall by the wayside. If you're lucky, this will last a few months.

Let's call this Honeymoon phase.

After the Honeymoon phase comes the Balance phase. This is the phase where you begin to remember what life was like before your partner, and how much you enjoyed your hobbies and activities. A little bit of separation ensues, anxiety sometimes included, and it's time that you leave your honeymoon sphere to re-enter the real world and how you can balance your relationship within it.

You juggle your priorities, tinker with your time management, and arrive at the balance of how much time you can devote to each other for the relationship. As you can imagine, a lot of conflicts follow because expectations are either upheld or unmet. This phase can make or break many couples, as it's a return from a fantasy world that isn't always representative of reality.

Next, we hit the Comfort phase. Zero effort put forth into cultivating or growing the relationship? Check. A slow de-prioritization of your partner? Check. Growing indifference to your partner's needs and desires?

Check. Apathy towards what your partner thinks of you? Check.

Weekends where you don't change out of your sweatpants? Check and double check.

The comfort and security that we hold in our relationships causes us to lose the motivation to maintain the person that your partner became attracted to in the first place. Ever hear of relationship weight? It's the same phenomenon. (On the other hand, it speaks to how amazing a motivator being single and not having access to sex is!)

The Comfort phase is where so many relationships tend to languish and die a slow death. And it runs both ways. What happened to the girl you fell in love with? For that matter, what happened to the guy *she* fell in love with?

(The next phases of course are the Tolerance phase and the Begrudgingly Still Together out of Obligation or Fear of Change phase... but this is neither the place nor time to discuss those.)

Did any of those descriptions resonate with you or perhaps make you cringe? That's what this book is about.

You'll learn how to become the type of man that keeps her woman captivated to recapture those intense feelings of desire and respect she held for you in the Chase, Honeymoon, or even Balance phase. You'll also learn how to build a deeper, stronger, and more fulfilling relationship with your woman in ways you never thought possible. Your relationship deserves those on a daily basis, and you shouldn't settle for anything less.

How can you break out of your slowly fading Comfort phase to ensure that your woman will continue to date and court you like it's still the Chase phase, and clamor for you to commit to her?

It's going to be a matter of resetting habits and patterns that may be hard-coded in you and your woman's mind, but the payoff will be worth it. You will learn how to inspire and motivate each other to new heights, and stand as two titans instead of one interdependent spire. You will understand how to embrace each other's vulnerabilities on a deep level.

And perhaps the ultimate payoff? There are going to be tell-tale signs throughout as to whether she's going to be the one or not, and I've also developed a series of powerful and revealing questions to evaluate her with.

Here's to building the strongest relationship of your life!

# 1. Being assertive isn't being an asshole.

"Asshole" is a term that most men (and people...) want to avoid like the plague.

There are just a host of negative connotations that come with it, and let's face it, they are sometimes true.

But work and relationship contexts aside, the worst part of the term "asshole" is the way that women use it to describe a man that takes charge and isn't afraid to offend others with his opinions. It's almost as if assertive is interchangeable with asshole at times, and it's a shame.

But I'm here to tell you that there are zero absolutely differences between being assertive and an asshole, and that you should never be afraid to be assertive and have your opinion heard.

I've met far too many men that simply don't like confrontation or to rock the boat – that's a dangerous slippery slope because it can be so gradual that you eventually find yourself mute in the relationship.

Wait, since when is it being an asshole to just say what's on your mind, or even what your preferences might be?

Assholes prod and provoke to make a point, which are often punctuated by emotional outbursts and accusations. Women have no issues responding to logic, so if you approach them on that level in an assertive manner, you will have their attention, respect, and never be called an asshole.

Assholes also tend to make points that aren't related to the actual point, which is mostly a matter of twisting the knife that they can sometimes wield. Not pleasant.

Tell me what you think women like: a passive man who bends to her every whim and is essentially whipped... or a strong man that isn't a doormat, who forces them to respect them, can take charge when necessary, and can be equals with them. Hint: it's not the first one.

So embrace assertiveness, because it is easy to do so without being a raging asshole.

# 2. Tarzan usually leads.

Men instinctually know that women want a man who leads. It's what every movie and Disney prince portrays, and it's not a stretch to say that our modern conception of romance and chivalry comes from popular media.

Even the high-powered female CEO wouldn't mind taking a backseat in her relationship at times, if only to give her mind a break from her demanding job. If you have to lead a relationship constantly, it's just draining and another source of work... not quite what you hope to get out of being with someone.

Gender roles aside, many women also instinctually want a man like this – however, they may not allow or give their man an opportunity to actually lead. They will either take the reins themselves, or shoot down the man's relatively subtle attempts to lead in favor of doing things their own way. It's a process that is like the Grand Canyon forming – it starts slowly, and you don't even notice that it's happening... until surely enough, you've taken the reins over from him and are planning out your weekends unilaterally.

So having this knowledge of what women desire… lead like men do, and don't let her take those reins! Be primitive and dominant Tarzan. Take charge and plan outings. To get her to play her part, don't be afraid to suggest that she fulfill the role of being the woman that you can take care of. These women appeal to his sense of animal masculinity and dominance and encourage him to bring it out. You will be surprised at how she will embrace that role if you embrace yours.

So more often than not, take hold of the reins and be the one to kill her spiders, open her jars, and be her Prince Charming in all ways possible. Feeling needed is a big part of the masculine drive for men in a relationship. We know that we're supposed to assume that role, and when we do, a whole other side of sexy dominance will come out. Once you feel the rush of taking control, you will embrace it like you never thought possible.

You will also never have to question if you are whipped, and it will restore the perceived balance of power in the relationship, which is powerful.

# 3. No time machines allowed during arguments.

It's a greater temptation than inhaling all of those donuts in the breakroom the moment no one is watching.

Bringing up the past in an argument? It's like a trump card, a doomsday device that simply obliterates the rest of the argument and ends it right there.

Except that the underlying issue is still lurking, and you've just uncovered old feelings of resentment... So now you're dealing with two issues where there was one before... and a much bigger chance of an emotional outburst from either of you.

Here's the thing.

Issues from old arguments have hopefully been settled, and they are almost always irrelevant to the actual issue at hand. So why even bring it up? There are a few reasons that people do this, men and women included.

First, they bring up old issues to try to "win" an argument that they sense they are losing.

Second, to obscure the facts of the issue at hand.

Third, because they are confused about the issue at hand.

None of those reasons actually contribute to solving the real issue at hand, and digging into the past is typically an emotional argument that concerns itself with baggage, and nothing more. A theme with those reasons is also that the person that is digging into the past is simply trying to prove that they are right... and what kind of reason is that to argue? That's the very definition of counterproductive.

Keep your argument focused on the present, because while the past does inform who you are, you both are different people now and should operate in that context.

# 4. Men can be "crazy" too.

I know that you feel what you feel, and no one should disregard that.

Trust me, I have 2 sisters who tell me the same on a weekly basis. No matter how irrational your feelings are, they are still valid and a reflection of your mental and emotional state. I get that.

But this is a chapter about reasonableness.

You can suddenly feel sadness wash over you if a dog crosses your path that resembles the pup you grew up with. That's reasonable.

But there's a lot of unreasonable reactions you might have in relation to your woman and her doings. Shall we dispel some of them? Her hanging out with her male friends alone or late at night. Going out with them. Not always wanting to have sex. Not always being in a great mood. Watching reality TV shows and obsessing over shopping. The list goes on.

Now before you get all up in arms against me, just realize that I'm not telling you that you're necessarily wrong or being an unreasonable person.

I'm just suggesting that you recognize the difference between your subjective reasonableness, and the objective reasonableness that the rest of the world operates on.

I'm not telling you which is correct or judging you on it – I'm just telling you that this is how your woman thinks and feels, so isn't it better to have that awareness?

To find your measure of subjective and objective reasonableness, simply turn to the peanut gallery that is your friends. And no, not just those pals who will agree with and support you to the ends of the earth. Get opinions from both genders, don't leave factors out just to make yourself look more in the right, and attempt to leave defensiveness behind.

You feel what you feel, and you are entitled to that, but that doesn't mean that it's always reasonable for you to act on it and expect others to conform to it. That's called entitlement.

# 5. Make it safe for her to be vulnerable.

A major part of an ace relationship is fostering an environment that is both welcoming and safe for all kinds of communication.

The moment that either you or your woman feels uncomfortable sharing things with the other is the moment that miscommunications arise, resentment starts festering, and the relationship is weakened.

Realize the following two things about yourself as a man: you have likely been taught to suppress vulnerability and emotional displays for your whole life, and you have been urged to be stoic and strong in front of the women that you are committing yourself to. Women, on the other hand, have been taught to suppress their sexual urges and libido... but that's another story.

Those are the hurdles that you are fighting when you seek to open up your vulnerabilities to your woman. But just because your woman hasn't been conditioned as you have been, doesn't mean that it's easy for her or anyone to truly open up and make themselves vulnerable. It's a scary process, so anytime anyone actually lets you in, appreciate her actions and take them as a sign of how strongly she feels about you.

So when you dig and dig and finally are able to squeeze something out of her, make it known that you are very accepting of those insecurities. Celebrate them and tell her how those very things make her more attractive to you and maybe even drew you to her in the first place.

Compliment her on them and make it a goal to raise her self-esteem about the very things she is self-conscious about. You'll see a new woman once you are able to connect over these issues – divulge some of your own to keep encouraging her and make her feel bonded to you.

The big disclaimer I have to give is that you have to know when you can push your woman and when to let off. She may already be in an inherently foreign and unnatural state of mind, and could feel violated if you push for too much too soon. That's a hurdle that you simply cannot bowl over, and only comes with time and increased comfort and security in the relationship that you are cultivating.

# 6. Match up your styles of affection.

Just as conflict styles, eating styles, and sleeping styles need to be aligned, you must learn to align your styles of showing and receiving affection with your woman.

The first step is recognizing that people actually show and receive love and affection in different ways! For some, this is a jarring realization that some of their biggest romantic gestures have fallen on deaf (or more accurate, apathetic) ears.

If you think you've been under-appreciated or taken for granted, it could be an effect of the phenomenon that your styles of affection haven't matched. And if you feel that you have been egregiously taken for granted, chances are that logically, your woman isn't taking you for granted... it's that your styles of affection don't match whatsoever.

So instead of having to read between the lines with every potentially sweet (or insensitive) act by your woman, it will be helpful to examine the typical framework that Gary Chapman describes in his research.

He describes 5 typical classifications of how people show and receive affection.

Physical touch, spending quality time together, spontaneous acts of kindness, words of affirmation, and performing their duties for them.

Most of these classifications are self-explanatory, but we can run through an example to see where a miscommunication can occur.

You feel that because your woman doesn't initiate sex with you very frequently, that she is distant and losing interest in you. However, your woman hasn't been initiating sex with you because she's been so tired from balancing your checkbook for you. You are valuing physical touch while she shows her affection through acts of kindness – not necessarily a mismatch, but definitely a miscommunication.

The recognition that affection can be shown in many ways might help you appreciate your woman more, and vice versa, especially when viewing the past through that lens.

# 7. Compromise, don't sacrifice.

Think for a second, if you can, about what drew you to your woman in the first place.

Her hair. Her buttocks probably.

I bet another essential aspect was that she was passionate about something, and pursued it outside of work with a burning passion and drive. After all, when someone is engaged, they become engaging.

So keeping in mind that your woman having a separate identity and passion was attractive... don't ask her to sacrifice either for the sake of your relationship. Don't make her choose between her priorities, habits, hobbies, friends... or anything else she used to spend her time on before she started dating you. If you force her to choose, you might win most of the time, but you won't like the consequences or what that means.

If she consistently begins to choose you over her other priorities, she will become more dependent on you than ever before. And when someone is dependent on you, it causes you to lose your independence as well because you will feel responsible for her happiness, obligated to spend time with her, and guilty if you don't.

It's not a good look for a relationship, nor is it healthy.

Because of that, she will also probably become flat out less attractive to you. Who sacrifices their other priorities and doesn't have a strong sense of self? It's just human nature that when people have other priorities, we automatically assume that they have so much more going on for them than those who do not. This assumption will be tough to overcome.

Finally, eventually your woman will grow a sense of resentment at not partaking in her favorite hobbies and passions. She will believe that she is making the choice himself every time to see you instead, but that doesn't mean she still won't blame you for it on some subconscious level.

If she is resentful, she will likely try to assert control or dominance in the relationship in some other way, which can be dangerous to deal with.

So allow – nay, enforce – space, and seize your own. When you take your own space and pursue your own passions, she can either sit there twiddling her thumbs waiting for you to return, or follow suit.

The best part is that if you give her this space to do what she wants without any type of guilt, she will feel lucky that you are so accommodating and you will forever be the "cool and chill" boyfriend.

# 8. Why can't you be more like Alison?

Women and insecurity. Kind of a duh statement, right?

We men certainly have our hangups and things in life that we are self-conscious about – do we not bleed? Do we not cry? Oh, we cry. Watching the Lion King will do that to anyone.

But it'd probably be a stretch to say that men are as insecure as women.

Therefore, even if you think a borderline statement wouldn't bother you… it could very well ruin your woman's day.

One of the worst that will undoubtedly eat away at your woman is comparing her to another woman. Compare her to Adriana Lima? Sure, go nuts – she'll probably agree with you that her curves are the epitome of the ideal woman.

But compare her to someone you both know, and you're going to have a bad time... especially when it's about something feminine or what Stephanie does for her boyfriend. And if you compare your current woman to your ex? Why wouldn't you just punch her in the ovaries to save time?

This will have several consequences that you may not have thought through.

First, it will cause her to feel inadequate because you're holding her to a standard that may not be fair or even logical.

Second, it will cause her to feel resentment towards the person that you both know, souring or preventing a friendship from forming because of it.

Third, her insecurities just became that much more concrete because it's someone tangible and real as opposed to Adriana Lima or Kate Upton.

You should think carefully about the reason you're even making a comparison. It might be an offhand comment, or you might want to make a point... but you're opening Pandora's Box of insecurities just to make that point. Couldn't it be made in a less inflammatory and more measured manner?

Let's just imagine what kind of tables you'd flip if your woman offhandedly compared you in a negative light to her ex, one of your best guy friends, or one of her male co-workers.

Being compared to Brad Pitt you're probably fine with, but when it's someone tangible, blood begins to boil.

# 9. Really, her favorite bands are a dealbreaker?

Let me preface this chapter with a simple proposition.

Very few of us have very legitimate dealbreakers when it comes to our partners. Sure, we all undoubtedly have laundry lists of things that we would like for them to be or embody... but not having those traits is almost never a dealbreaker.

Religion, whether they desire children, whether they engage in recreational drug use, if they are a swinger, and chemistry. Those are most of the real dealbreakers that exist for any couple.

Most anything else? Yes, they are just preferences.

The easiest way to tell the difference between your preferences and real dealbreakers is to actually start dating someone... because chances are that once you meet someone and like them already, most things you thought you cared about don't really matter that much as long as you have chemistry with her.

This is a process that can take years for us to discover. We can either go the route of finding out from date to date and relationship to relationship what really matters or us, or we can dig deep into introspection... either way, this is a powerful realization that should cause you to at least examine what you've been searching for in your woman, and why that is.

You might cycle through what you thinks matters but doesn't. What you think *should* matter but doesn't. What others have pressured you into thinking matters, but doesn't. What your mom tells you that matters, but doesn't.

Knowing yourself and what you want is a lifelong journey, but beginning to realize what your preferences are and what your real dealbreakers are can save you a lot of time, effort, and ultimately heartache by finding a woman that fits you snugly without the burden of expectations.

# 10. Rationalization is usually a cover.

Rationalization is usually an exercise in allowing oneself to avoid the truth of a matter, and justifying something that isn't acceptable... into acceptability.

We can look at some of the more common ones before diving deep into how this affects you and your relationship with your woman.

While dieting, you decide that it's okay to splurge on a baker's dozen of chocolate glazed donuts because you've worked hard in the gym for the past day and therefore deserve a cheat meal.

While at Disneyland, you decide that it's okay to buy a t-shirt that costs $80 because who knows the next time you'll be there, and you want a souvenir!

While in bumper to bumper gridlock traffic, you decide that it's okay to scream and flip the bird to every car around you while blasting Miley Cyrus.

Some of those are more acceptable than others, of course.

And you with your woman?

While she makes fun of you when you're out together with friends, you decide that it's okay because she's just joking around and trying to impress your friends.

While she doesn't clean up or contribute to the household chores at all, you decide that it's okay because she's tired and had a long day at work.

My point here is that you shouldn't rationalize her actions or find yourself in the position to make excuses for her behavior. If it's bad, it's objectively bad, circumstances notwithstanding. No excuses or buts.

It's also important to think about the psychology of why someone would continue to make excuses for their woman – is it because there is a speck inside them that believes that they deserve the treatment that they get? Does it speak to their self-esteem and self-worth?

I can't tell you which end of the spectrum you fall on, but this should definitely be food for thought.

# 11.  Who loves you the most? You!

Remember those friends you used to have that completely disappeared once they got into relationships? How did you feel about that vanishing act?

Probably negatively, to say the least.

You wanted your friend back, but you also felt that your friend was losing parts of his individual identity and slowly becoming a Frankenstein of her and him. Jonathan and Cathy? Nope, there's only Jonathy now.

But really, the biggest problem that these friends (or you...) have is that they have made themselves dependent on their woman for their happiness, and that they don't feel complete without her. Fairy tales aside, this is an extremely unhealthy approach to a relationship for a number of reasons.

First, you lose your identity and probably many of the reasons that your woman became attracted to you in the first place.

Second, you run the big risk of becoming a burden to your woman, because when you become dependent on her, you make her lose her own independence because she will feel obligated to spend more time with you, and feel guilt when she does not. You will become that ball and chain.

The solution here is not as actionable as other points have been, but there's a specific mindset tweak you must apply.

You are responsible for your own happiness... she's undoubtedly a part of that, but only a part, and doesn't act to complete you.

She obviously needs to be made a priority, but too many men skew the other way and figuratively prostrate themselves to their women – and wonder why their women grow bored and restless at the lack of a challenge.

In summation, your life is vibrant on its own, and she is but an addition to it... like a sunroof to a car.

# 12. Inspire her, motivate her.

Before we talk about being her muse, let's gather some context by talking about the opposite of a muse – a parasite.

A parasite latches itself onto an unsuspecting host and lives off of the host, depending on it utterly for sustenance and life. It adds literally nothing to the host's life and existence, and even weakens the host. Finally, a parasite will wither away to nothing and die if separated from the host.

Now imagine how many men you know that turn into said parasites when they into relationships with their women (hosts). In hindsight or on the perch of an objective observer, maybe you yourself have been guilty of acting the parasite!

This chapter is about the anti-parasite – the muse. Instead of dragging her down and putting your dependence on her, act as your woman's muse by seeking to inspire, enlighten, and motivate her.

A truly healthy relationship should act as a vehicle towards self-growth and development with your woman. Ideally, a couple develops together and continues to find new ways to enrich their lives... but this isn't possible if either party is a parasite. Adding value simply isn't possible from a dependent party.

Inspiring and motivating starts with you – you must actively become her muse. This is a process that begins with you and your lifestyle. When you set expectations for yourself and surpass them, your woman will follow suit and step up to the plate to equal you. When you pursue your own passions diligently and hotly, she will take note and be encouraged to pursue her own. When you have a thirst for adventure and life, she can't help but feel challenged in the best way possible. If she doesn't do any of the above, you might have a problem on your hands.

It all comes down to how you envision your happy relationship looking like. Do you seek a balance of minds that contributes to mutual growth and development?

Once you ensure that you yourself are challenging and inspiring, you can impart the rest to your woman.

# 13. The only "The One" questions you'll need.

You can pick up any issue of Maxim or other so-called men's magazines and you'll get simply inundated with criteria for what your future wife should encompass.

She's got to have a great mother-in-law, a wonderful head of hair, and an earning potential of at least six figures. Barring that, she must be tirelessly dedicated to her craft and passion, or a gentle soul and potentially amazing mother.

Doesn't have those? Then she better have an amazing set of sweater puppies and stems.

Not saying that those things don't matter... But on the whole as criteria for evaluating your future wife? Let's take a step back and really focus on the things that matter. Hint – it's a lot simpler than it's made out to be.

First, do you feel challenged by your woman?

A relationship, as I've touched on before, shouldn't be a static creature. A healthy relationship grows each year, and develops into a more deep connection and bond with each other. The way you relate to each other will also change, as you grow personally and yet closer to each other in the same direction. Yet growth won't occur if you don't feel challenged by your woman to keep improving. Your woman should be your best cheerleader and inspire and motivate you to be the best version of yourself. Staying at the same level of growth is eventually going to be the same as no growth at all.

Second, do you respect your woman?

Regardless of which camp you are in with respect – whether it must be earned, or whether it is given freely and deducted as a result of actions and intentions – respect has the tendency to wane and wither without proper attention.

No one deserves respect unconditionally (sans perhaps your parents), and the level at which we respect people should gradually rise or decrease. Do your respect your woman's career, morals, intentions, life habits, hobbies, and choices? It doesn't necessarily mean that you have to like her choices, but respect is a different animal altogether.

Finally, is she, or does she have the potential to be your best friend?

It turns out that relationships, after the sparks and chemistry die off slowly, are about the friendship you form with your woman. The day to day aspects about the other person that make you laugh and love them. This might be the least surprising part of this chapter to focus on, but it still needs to be said.

Your woman ideally should be one of your best friends – your favorite person in the world, regardless of if you were having sex with her. The one you want to spend the most time with, and the one you can sit around in sweatpants on weekends and feel perfectly content and entertained with.

In case the answers to those three big ones are hazy (they usually are...), here are some ancillary questions that I've found helpful to frame people with.

Does she bring out the best in you? Make you want to be a better person? Does she make the ordinary or mundane seem acceptable or extraordinary? Does she comfort you and make you feel safe? Do you feel lucky to be with her?

So Maxim be damned, it's time to re-examine what our priorities really are!

# 14. Day to day chemistry beats the rich yoga instructor.

Yup, this is a point that bears repeating. It's a somewhat different thesis from the previous chapter, and focuses a bit more on what draws you to your woman in the first place.

What really matters when you're evaluating whether your woman is relationship material, and ultimately is in it to win it (for marriage)?

I'll tell you what isn't important: her sexy body, if she is loaded financially, where she went to school, what her parents do, where she grew up, what her favorite bands are, what she likes to do in her free time, what instruments she plays, what her earning potential is, what sports she plays, how much she hikes, and whether she is an Apple fangirl or not.

However you envision your life and relationship unfolding, those are simply unfounded expectations and fantasies that do their best to disrupt reality time and time again.

If the day to day chemistry is there, you'll figure the rest out and make it work, won't you?

Which brings me to my main point. The day to day of a relationship is the part that truly matters and makes you happy and fulfilled. That's when you truly love someone for who they are, as opposed to becoming enamored with how they fit together on paper and the idea of who they are.

Depending on the big picture stuff – the same things I did not espouse earlier, like education, school, parents, sports, hobbies – they are important. Don't get that twisted, clearly some of those things matter.

But depending on them to cement or carry a relationship while ignoring the day to day, well that's just a recipe for a an incredibly unsatisfying relationship and a middle-aged divorce where we'll all bemoan having to date again *at our age*! Simply put, they are meaningless without conversational and romantic chemistry that lasts beyond the honeymoon period.

Your woman is going to be your partner, so beyond the chemistry, you also need to be able to connect with them over just about everything in your life, feel comfortable being vulnerable and opening up to them, resolve issues and conflicts in a healthy manner, and simply enjoy them.

I think we can all admit that the former college cheerleader and yoga instructor automatically has a leg up on others initially (literally), but it's important to realize that that allure is going to be very fleeting if you can't connect with her on deeper levels.

# 15. "Maybe" is usually "I'm scared to actually say no."

I believe that at their core, people do not change.

Barring some life-flashing-before-my-eyes situation, people are who they are by the time you get into a relationship with them. Their outlooks, style of conflict, and perception of what a relationship encompasses are all static and mostly immutable.

I realize that many of you will disagree with me on that assertion, but allow me to explain how it ties into the thesis of this chapter.

It's a situation we've all encountered at some point or another:

"So do you love her/want to marry her/see this going long-term?"

"Maybe..."

Well, here's the thesis.

"Maybe" typically means "I'm too scared to actually say no right now..." when deep inside, you know that things probably won't change for the better in order for your "Maybe" to turn into a "Yes" or even a "Probably."

I believe most of you can relate to and agree with this assertion.

In the context of a relationship, people have their patterns, and it usually takes an Armageddon-esque event for things to truly change. You'll have an argument about her not showing enough affection or refusing to spend time with you and your friends when you go out... and things may change for about 3 weeks.

But next time it comes up, she'll be back to her old habits, figuring she's out of the doghouse.

That's not a change, that's just *appeasement*.

Now what about bigger issues, such as whether someone wants children, where they see themselves ending up, or living with one's parents and extended family? These are real issues, and people may not ever change their stances on them.

You can't go into a relationship hoping that things will change your way... which means that your "maybe" might be a tacit and instinctual understanding of that.

If you're 2 years into a relationship and it's a maybe, examine whether you really want to say no and what exactly is preventing you from doing so. It's no one's fault that people are wired the way that they are, but an important skill in life is to know when to cut your losses and accept that things won't magically improve after your next milestone. As with many things, simply realizing this is only a tiny sliver of the battle, and the pulling the trigger is everything else.

But at some point if it's not a slam dunk, far too much rationalization is happening in the background, and it's probably a no.

# 16. Relationship pants are meant for two.

Ever have those days where work was a bitch, the coffee maker backfired, and you somehow got stuck in bumper to bumper traffic?

I bet you just want to get home, take your pants and shoes off (in that order), and collapse into your couch with a beer and a steak.

And then your woman gets home, asks what you want for dinner, and what you want to do Friday night.

Now imagine that happening every night. Tiring, isn't it? So don't do that to your woman!

This isn't a chapter about being decisive or planning ahead. It's about being an active participant in the relationship, and not making your woman make all of the decisions. In other words, don't put her in your shoes from above.

Before you unequivocally state that you don't do this, just imagine how many times you've used the phrase "I don't know/care, you decide."

For God's sake, just decide where to eat once in a while. And not just in the "I don't care, but not x, y, z, a, b, or c. Anything else is fine."

I realize that many men are fine with the traditional gender roles of taking charge and embracing the relationship pants... but many other men just don't have an opinion about such things.

But now that you've seen things from the other side – you're tired from a long day of work, probably cranky, and now you have to keep dealing with the mental burden of making decisions instead of being able to shut your brain off?

What value is your woman getting out of your relationship if she has to direct everything and take on the mental burden of doing that?

First of all, it's just boring to deal with someone that has no opinion at all.

Second, it gets old very quickly, having that kind of perceived power. Is it as drastic as I'm making it out to be? Of course not... initially. But it's a lazy answer and mindset that can invade every aspect of your relationship, which is why it's so dangerous.

If one of the subconscious reasons that you don't want to voice your opinion is to avoid taking a stance and continue people-pleasing, you can at the very least present choices!

My point here is to avoid being a passive participant in your relationship… because in what way is it a relationship then?

## 17. Let her feminine qualities shine.

Women are nothing if not their egos and insecurities.

It's not a stretch to say that having both of those is an essential part of the feminine identity, what with all the expectations of femininity and caretaking (if you prescribe to those traditional gender roles).

Given that, there are some aspects of your woman that you should take relative pity on, because it will do significantly more damage than it would otherwise. Even if your woman is as easygoing as a piece of pie, there are things that she is still especially sensitive about.

As the title reads, don't undermine her traditionally feminine and caretaking qualities.

What are traditional feminine qualities?

Qualities centered on nurturing, caretaking, providing, delicateness, being pretty, and curating. Besides those, traits that she prides herself on. The ones where if you take her duties away from her, she will feel inadequate and emasculated.

If you happen to be better than your woman at any of these things (and you probably are), feel free to downplay it or de-emphasize it lest you damage her ego and deflate her self-worth in the relationship.

Most women feel most comfortable when they are allowed to act the feminine part in a relationship, and if you take that away from her, you may cause her to overcompensate in other ways that will likely be detrimental to the relationship. Studies have shown time and time again that many men are uncomfortable with the prospect of being a stay-at-home father or earning less than their wives – and this is no different of a mindset.

If you let her fulfill what she perceives her duties to be, and every woman has different perceptions in different relationships, she will retain her self-esteem and channel that confidence back into the relationship with you.

## 18. She already has one father.

As I've alluded to a few times before, gender roles are still incredibly prevalent in our society. They're not always detrimental, and can sometimes help us organize and understand.

In many ways, gender roles are directly tied to our modern day conception of romance. Chivalry. The Damsel in Distress. The Caretaker. The Defender.

However, all of those roles are predicated on treating your woman in the way that a man treats his mate... and not in the way that a father treats his daughter.

You must straddle the line between your protective instincts, and smothering father territory.

Fathering has the distinct effect of making someone feel smothered and that they are being tracked for someone else's purposes... and how exactly did you react to your parent that was like that? At the very least, annoyed. At worst, wanting to break free and get far, far away.

She'll feel cornered and instantly look for an escape route. Like the daughter of an overbearing father, she may even rebel against you and lash out in ways you might not anticipate.

Not the effect that you want to create in your woman, but that's what happens when you treat her like a daughter/inmate.

This isn't a chapter about avoiding clinginess; rather, it's about avoiding the urge to constantly check in, nag, direct her activities, lecture, preach, and accommodate.
Even if your relationship with your woman is as healthy as an ox, and she doesn't mind the excessive amount of attention and doting, you create a negative association with each of your interactions. She will feel obligated to spend time with you, and may even do so sometimes out of guilt.

You're putting your expectations on someone else, and anytime that happens, they will feel burdened to have to live up to them.

Again, a sense of guilt or duty being the reason that your woman spends time with you?

Not ideal.

# 19.  Exes are like Seal Team 6.

By the time you hit your late 20's, it's unavoidable that people come into relationships and even dates with a bit of baggage.

The amount of baggage I carry in my late 20's for me might even be the equivalent of early 20's for some... and late 30's for others!

People develop at different rates, but my underlying point is that no matter how hard you try, you're going to have a lot of difficulty finding someone without a history of exes and the associated baggage.

Not all baggage is negative, and I don't mean to use the word in that way – rather, baggage is simply pre-conceived notions, assumptions, and habits that people carry with them into their next relationships as a result of their past. This is perfectly expected and never a negative reflection of yourself.

Which brings me to the biggest piece of baggage, and the title of this chapter.

Exes. Treat them like Seal Team 6 (the Seal Team that killed Osama Bin Laden). Only disclose about them on a need to know basis, and even then, be careful about what gets into the open.

No sexual details. Stay within generalities. DON'T COMPARE HER TO YOUR EX.

There are really only a few reasons for your exes to come up in conversation, and there are even fewer legitimate reasons. Sure, sometimes they inform who we are and what we do, but more often than not, the topic of exes only arises to satisfy curiosities that are better left unspoken.

And when you find out something that you'd rather not have known? Jealousy. Inadequacy. Insecurity. All of the emotions that you thought you had in check can come tumbling out if you find out something that just happens to strike a chord of your biggest insecurities.

Talking about the baggage of exes will result in drama more often than you would see the fruits of any benefit reaped, which is why I always recommend treating them like Seal Team 6.

The past is the past, and it's more important to be present and accept someone for who they are at that moment. The person that really learns from the past is the one who went through it – you don't need to know those parts about your woman... because she'll show them to you in due time.

# 20.  Why doesn't she just "want sex more"?

Throughout this book, I've often alluded to the fact that we men are less emotionally open, vulnerable, and perceptive. Women of course are less sexually expressive, desiring, and generally open.

The annoying part about this is that there is a near-complete overlap between those lacking traits, and what each sex feels is lacking from their ideal relationships.

I don't necessarily believe that women are less sexual creatures inherently. Men are women aren't necessarily wired that differently. But they *are* brought up and socialized incredibly differently.

From childhood, men are taught to be stoic, tough, not show emotions, not cry, and to simply "man up" when a tough situation arises. If they aren't able to do so, it's a jab at their masculinity and very identity as a modern male. Emotional intimacy and vulnerable are weaknesses that must be hidden and covered up. At the same time, they are encouraged to be virile conquerors of women. So it's no wonder that men often have issues being vulnerable, even to the woman in their life.

Likewise, women from birth have been taught to suppress their sexuality, slut-shame, preserve false modesty, downplay their libidos, and otherwise act the part of "the lady." They are encouraged to open up emotionally to their friends, and socialize with empathy and sympathy.

Is there a mismatch here?

*The traits and attributes that men and women have been taught to desire the most is exactly what society has taught the other sex to suppress.*

This isn't a chapter about undoing years of gender role socialization.

Rather, it's about understanding exactly what you're up against when you ask your woman to simply "want sex more" and other such phrases. It's going against so many of her built in defense mechanisms, her upbringing, the years of potential ridicule and shaming from female friends. If you're able to get her to open up sexually in a free manner, it will likely be one of the first times she's ever done it, so you'll need to practice patience.

She's likely going to be amazingly out of her comfort zone, so you must cultivate a safe space for her to be sexually open with you.

This chapter might also serve to inform you about why women emphasize emotional intimacy so much, and why your signals to her can be frustrating – purely as a result of your socialization and upbringing.

## 21. Absence makes the heart (and other things) grow fonder.

We all know the feelings that arise after not seeing your significant other for a stretch of time — the longing, the missing, the increased libido...

Here's a dirty secret.

You can create that feeling of absence in more ways than you think, and absence doesn't have to exist purely from business trips or long-distance relationships.

The feeling of absence can take the place of a well-timed guy's night out, planning for a weekend away with your family...

But what's the common thread that creates an absence that will make your woman yearn for you?

Taking and owning your space away from her.

Making the conscious choice to spend time away from her, which has the funny effect of making her clamor to be your top priority time and time again. When you own your own space, you also give her her own space, which she will love you for.

You will become the "cool, chill boyfriend" that isn't clingy or possessive... and yet (ironically) she will begin to assert a kind of ownership over you that tells you that she misses you more, and cares about what you're doing and who you're seeing.

It's not a sense of jealousy, rather, it's a form of deference by her that acknowledges and respects your own life and happenings.

The reality is that when you are engaged in other things, you become that much more engaging yourself... and it will make her realize how much she misses you and wants to be around you.

Remember the reasons you were attracted to your woman in the first place – her passions, interests, and hobbies?

Preserve yours and make the heart grow fonder on a day-to-day basis.

## 22. It's okay to be selfish sometimes.

I hate the word "selfish."

It contains so many negative associations, and the word by itself is treated like a cancer.

But since when is it such a terrible thing to prioritize yourself above others?

Further, is it a terrible sin to do what makes you happy on a day-to-day basis and accept that the priorities of others are not as important as yours?

What about making you and your needs the center of your world and actions?

No, being selfish is not inherently a negative aspect, especially when it comes to relationships. I know that this sounds like the opposite of the advice you usually hear about how you should regard your woman, but bear with me. It's the curse of the slippery slope.

When you subordinate yourself to your woman and place all of her priorities above yours, what does your day-to-day look like? You do what she wants to do, you spend your time taking care of her and catering to her, and most importantly you leave no room for what is important to you.

In a sense, the relationship has taken you and your priorities hostage, and you will only see your priorities and hobbies alive again when the relationship ends!

So now that we're all operating in the same context, how does being selfish sound now? I think you'll find that "selfish" sometimes means just doing thing for yourself – which is necessary and central to a healthy balanced relationship.

Your woman is certainly a priority, but she may not even be your top priority for as long as we live in the real world and not a Disney-like fantasy. And her priorities and needs certainly shouldn't always cut the line before yours!

This is a chapter about avoiding being a people-pleaser, because people-pleasers tend to be taken advantage of, taken for granted, and be criminally under-appreciated. People-pleasers also tend to eschew their own needs, because they think that other people's priorities are more important than theirs.

Referring back to the title again: sometimes you must be selfish with your priorities, and realize that selfish is not always negative!

# 23.  A spark is easy, a fire is tough.

I'm clearly a fan of analogies, so here's the meaning behind the title of this chapter.

Initial chemistry, the electric spark, and the ensuing honeymoon period is one of the easiest things to accomplish.

It doesn't require any effort because you're not really living in the real world at that point. You're just riding a hormonal and emotional high at the prospect of finding someone that likes you as much as you like them, and it's a self-fueling infatuation cycle.

And then reality hits. Work starts to ramp up. The infatuation wears off.

You remember that you have other friends that want to see you. Wait, didn't you used to play guitar?

And thus the spark has gone out. But what about the fire – that lasting love that fuels thriving relationships?

How can you still capture that with your woman while you're out of the honeymoon phase?

Unsurprisingly, it comes down to effort and really committing to growing you and your woman's fire.

So how can you channel effort into the fire?

First, recall how you went out of your way to see her and do little things for her, just to see how she would react. Well, do some of those things! If her appreciation doesn't do it for you, then rest assured knowing that sometimes when we act, our minds justify those actions – if I did this for Cathy, then I must be in love with her!

Second, routine is death for a relationship. It's the hallmark of a lack of effort and being resigned to a status quo that may or may not be fulfilling. So generate spontaneity, even if you have to plan it! You clearly enjoy spending time with your woman, so why not spend time with her in new and exciting places and events? Don't live your relationship on the couch of your apartment – remember how exciting it was to explore and share the world with her!

Finally, when you're used to something or someone, you eventually stop taking notice of the little things that they do for you. They just become invisible because you are so accustomed to it. That's not positive, and it's a shortcut to saying that things have been taken for granted.

Take a step back, and try to really document all the things that your woman does for you. Thank her profusely, and praise her on her own life and accomplishments. Chances are, that praise is incredibly under-utilized.

We all start somewhere, but it's a matter of making effort on a day-to-day and even moment-to-moment that can change the entire tone of a relationship into a white-hot blaze.

# 24. Fear the routine.

I touched upon this in the previous chapter, but breaking the daily humdrum routine of your relationship is one of the most effective steps in maintain a fulfilling partnership.

For some, this means spending some time apart and being able to appreciate what their partner brings into their life.

For some, this means going out together with to re-discover why you enjoyed spending so much time together in the first place.

For some, this means trying to fuse two different hobbies together so they can both indulge in each other's lives.

And yet for others, this means experimenting sexually.

Just as the relationship spark needs to be re-lit periodically into a powerful, slow-burning fire, so does what constitutes your routine.

A routine is not always negative, but it frequently leads to boredom in a relationship and with each other, which causes each party to seek excitement and varying degrees of fulfillment outside of the relationship. To be sure, elements of this are normal and expected. But there comes a tipping point when the routine is suffocating and an obligation rather than something to be looked forward to.

So how can you break routines routinely?

It's all about putting forth the effort into examining where you can inject excitement into the routine and continue to explore each other's personalities. Take an improv class together, volunteer together, go camping together, or re-model your home together.

It will cause you to see your woman (and vice versa) in an entirely new light, and reveal different aspects of his personality that you didn't even know existed... because you never bothered looking for them or allowed those parts to shine through.

Recognize also that many women are content to fulfill the traditional gender role of remaining passive and may expect the man to do all of the courting and work. This should act to encourage you to action, because though breaking routines takes two, you need to start somewhere! In the end, she'll appreciate you that much more for actively caring and putting the effort in. (The alternative being that she will resent you for not putting any effort in).

And that prior comfortable routine? It'll still be there when you come back, and you just might gain some things to add to it that will be hugely beneficial for your relationship's long-term health.

# Conclusion

Let's review our relationship phases. Chase, Honeymoon, Balance, and Comfort.
It is my sincerest hope that you now understand what it takes to stay in whichever phase that you wish – likely a mix of all the above! But above all to remain out of the Comfort phase for the good and health of your relationship.

It is equal parts elevating yourself to be the kind of man that your woman is captivated by, and dealing with specific relationship and partnership issues in ways to command commitment and heighten attraction.

Some of these principles are counterintuitive, but I implore you to let them sink in and re-visit this book at a later point. It is the culmination of years of relationship coaching, and I wish nothing for the most beneficial effects for you.

How do you keep her captivated? It turns out that common sense isn't always so common, but now you can be the bedrock in any relationship or even friendship you possess.

Your life will improve immensely as your relationships grow and mature, and after all... what else is there in life?

Sincerely,
Patrick King
Dating and Image Coach
www.thealphaworks.com

P.S. If you enjoyed this book, please don't be shy and drop me a line, leave a review, or both! I love reading feedback, and reviews are the lifeblood of Kindle books, so they are always welcome and greatly appreciated.

Other books by Patrick King include:

Why Women Love Jerks: Realizing the Best Version of Yourself to Effortlessly Attract Women
http://www.amazon.com/dp/B00KLPXNI0

CHATTER: Small Talk, Charisma, and How to Talk to Anyone

http://www.amazon.com/dp/B00J5HH2Y6

Charm Her Socks Off: Creating Chemistry from Thin Air

http://www.amazon.com/dp/B00IEO688W

# Cheat Sheet

Inside Her (Mind): Secrets of the Female Psyche to Attract Women, Keep Them Seduced, and Bulletproof Your Relationship

Introduction

1.      Being assertive isn't being an asshole. Assholes play with emotions and prod and provoke, while assertive and dominant men simply aren't afraid to state their mind.

2.      Tarzan usually leads. Take the lead in your relationship like society and your women probably expect and prefer.

3.      No time machines allowed during arguments. Don't bring up issues form the past and inject them into current arguments.

4.      Men can be "crazy" too. You are entitled to your opinion and perspective, but realize that that doesn't mean other people should share it or accommodate it.

5.     Make it safe for her to be vulnerable. Create a space for your woman to share her insecurities with you and strive to turn them into things she is proud about.

6.     Match up your styles of affection. Everyone has different love languages and it can be immensely helpful to discover which you are your woman are.

7.     Compromise, don't sacrifice. Let your woman keep his own priories and hobbies, because those are what drew you to her in the first place.

8.     Why can't you be more like Alison? Never compare your woman to another female that you both know, and especially never your ex.

9.     Really, her favorite bands are a dealbreaker? Examine if the traits you emphasize really matter to you, or if you just *think* they matter and have unfounded expectations surrounding them.

10.     Rationalization is usually a cover. If you find yourself constantly rationalizing and making excuses for your how you are treated by your woman, it's time to examine what that says about the level of respect in your relationship.

11.     Who loves you the most? You! A woman is like the sunroof of a car – great to have, but only a part of the overall package.

12. Inspire her, motivate her. Inspire and motivate your woman by first becoming someone inspiring and motivating yourself.

13. The only "The One" questions you'll need. Does she challenge you, do you respect her, and are you potentially best friends? Everything else is a wash.

14. Day to day chemistry beats the rich yoga instructor. What truly matters in a relationship is explosive chemistry and communication. Everything else on your laundry list of desired traits is simple a "nice to have."

15. "Maybe" is usually "I'm scared to actually say no." Examine the ones you are saying no to a commitment, and discover that there may be underlying reasons behind it.

16. Relationship pants are meant for two. Don't be a passive party and let your woman plan everything and dominate the interactions. She will get nothing out of the relationship.

17. Let her feminine qualities shine. Women have egos. Don't belittle their traditionally feminine qualities, traits, and skills.

18. She already has one father. There is a thin line between protecting and taking care of her... and fathering and nagging.

19.	Exes are like Seal Team 6. Do not mention exes except on a need to know basis, and control the spread of information whenever possible.

20.	Why doesn't she just "want sex more"? We men desire sexual openness and desire... too bad women have been taught to suppress their sexual urges since youth.

21.	Absence makes the heart (and other things) grow fonder. Taking your own space on a day to day basis, and making her take her own, will make her respect and desire you more.

22.	It's okay to be selfish sometimes. Don't let the relationship and your woman's priorities take over yours, because then you will lose yourself.

23.	A spark is easy, a fire is tough. Initial chemistry requires literally zero work, but stoking the relationship fire is all effort, all the time.

24.	Fear the routine. Routine is the bane of many relationships, so step outside your comfort zones and allow you and your woman to see each other in different lights.

Made in the USA
Columbia, SC
03 February 2021